THE NO-DIET DIET

INTERMITTENT FASTING GUIDE AND KETOGENIC TRICKS TO HEAL YOUR BODY AND UNLOCK STORED ENERGY

CONTENTS

Introduction

This book contains top secret information on how you can get in a better shape, heal your body and live a longer healthy life without dieting! Will you take the chance?

Intermittent fasting is not just another restricted calorie diet. There's plenty of those to go around. We're not about to offer you a rehashed version. As a matter of fact, intermittent fasting is not a diet at all.

Rather than a diet, intermittent fasting is an eating pattern. The pattern is divided into two alternating cycles. You have a period of feasting and a period for fasting. There is no list of food you are only allowed to eat. There is no need to change what kind of foods you eat. You can stick to the meals you are used to. The only thing you have to change is when you eat. In other words, you set a schedule for your meals in order to maximize what get out of them.

By consciously skipping meals, you can lose fat and build lean muscles. More importantly, it can help you heal your body and prevent diseases.

-You can reduce inflammation and oxidative stress.

-You can stimulate cellular repair processes.

-You can reduce your risk to diabetes.

-You can keep your circadian rhythm in sync and prevent metabolic diseases.

-You can reduce your risk to cardiovascular diseases.

-You can reduce your risk to cancer.

-You can prevent neurodegenerative diseases.

-You can promote better brain function.

-You can live longer!

Please be warned, this book contains a lot of spoilers that will possibly turn your world upside down!

Thanks for downloading this book, I hope you enjoy it!

Chapter 1
What's all the Fuss about Intermittent Fasting?

Do you want to lose weight? Go fasting! The mere mention of fasting scares people away. It really does conjure negative images. A lot of people would rather be picky with the things they eat but starvation is not something they are comfortable with.

When we're so used to hearing about how important breakfast is, being told otherwise can be quite a shock! When we are convinced that eating six small meals in a day is best for weight loss, it is natural to raise our eyebrows when we hear about fasting. After all, we need to be operating at our maximum throughout the day.

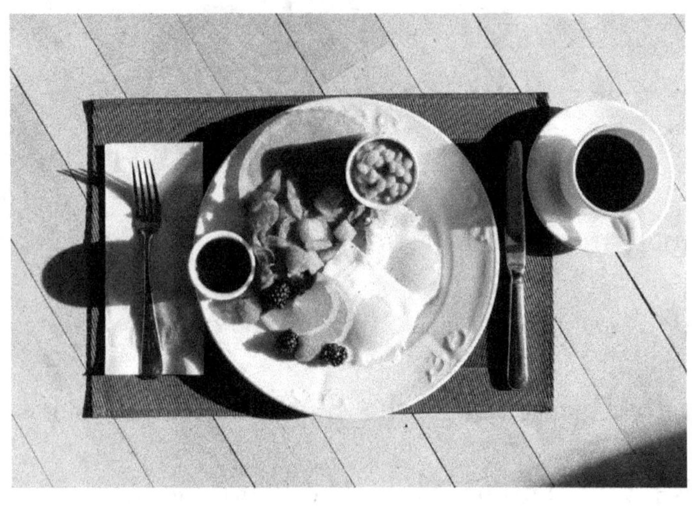

Breakfast like a king?

URL Source:

https://www.pexels.com/photo/food-gourmet-on-top-of-brown-table-101533/

Losing weight is not our job. So, we go on eating breakfast like a king, having lunch like a prince and taking dinner like a pauper. How's your diet working out for you? How many times have you started a diet that you quit after realizing just how unrealistic it is for your lifestyle?

What if skipping breakfast means losing weight, getting over that plateau while ensuring your optimum human performance? What if giving up the king's meal in the morning can mean physical and mental health improvement? What if not eating breakfast can offer your body fat loss and maximum muscle retention at the same time? Won't that be great? Indeed, it is! And it's exactly what intermittent fasting offers!

Intermittent Fasting is not a diet!

Let's clarify some things before we begin. First, intermittent fasting is not just another restricted calorie diet. There's plenty of those to go around. We're not about to offer you a rehashed version. As a matter of fact, intermittent fasting is not a diet at all.

Because intermittent fasting is not a diet, you do not have to count calories. You don't even need to weigh your food or measure them. You don't necessarily have to pick your food from a limited list. And you don't have to spend a lot of money buying foods "healthy" foods or setting aside time to figure out complicated recipes to abide by the strict rules of your diet.

Rather than a diet, intermittent fasting is an eating pattern. The pattern is divided into two alternating cycles. You have a period of eating and a period for fasting. There is no list of food you are only allowed to eat. There is no need to change what kind of foods you eat. You can stick to the meals you are used to. The only thing you have to change is when you eat. In other words, you set a schedule for your meals in order to maximize what get out of them.

To follow intermittent fasting, you have to consciously decide to skip certain meals during the day. You have to feast and fast on purpose. There is no need to count calories but you have to consume calories only during your period of eating which should be scheduled on a specific window on the day. And on the period of fasting, you should consciously choose not to eat on a larger time frame.

When to break your fast?

There are various methods of intermittent fasting that you can apply. These methods usually split the day or the week into a cycle of eating and fasting periods. So, intermittent fasting sounds great but you're probably wondering if you can fast and still function.

You may not realize it but the truth is, everybody fasts every single day. It happens when we sleep. You don't wake up in the middle of the night four hours after dinner to eat again. Unless you do then that makes you an exception. In any case, most of us fast from the time we have dinner until the time we wake up in the morning. This is why the first meal of the day is called such because it is meant to break your fast during the night. Intermittent fasting is simply extending the fast. For instance, instead of eating at 7am, they wait until lunch time for their first meal of the day for those who decide to skip breakfast.

You may think that's during the night when you have nothing to do but sleep. What happens when you don't have anything in the morning? How can you possibly function on an empty stomach? Well, many people don't seem to have a problem with this. It is not rocket science. It is simple and easy to follow. As a matter of fact, most people say the feel better and actually feel more energized during their period of fasting.

Of course, there is a feeling of hunger. And this can be a huge challenge especially in the beginning. But there is always difficulty when you are introducing a change. The body just needs some time to get used to the new routine.

Before you panic, it is not like taking a laboratory test where you need ten to twelve hours of fasting, from water included. We're not sadistic. In intermittent fasting, you are allowed to drink water during the fasting period. Insert sigh of relief. And if you happen to decide to skip breakfast which is the most common route, you can have either tea or coffee in the morning! Gasp. In fact, you are allowed to have any non-caloric beverage. There are other forms of IF that also allow little amounts of foods that are low in calorie during the period of fasting. Supplements are also allowed as long as there's zero calories in them.

We arc not the first to fast!

Although intermittent fasting has become a phenomenon in recent years, we are not the first to fast. Our ancestors have been doing it for thousands of years. They may have not thought to call it intermittent fasting or even cared to label what they're doing because fasting was just part of their routine. It probably wasn't because they wanted to lose weight. they fasted out of necessity. They didn't have a fridge before. They didn't have supermarkets. They had to hunt for food and when food isn't available, they had no choice but to wait for the next meal and cross their fingers for a lucky break.

Many religions also require fasting or some form of it. Muslims have to observe strict fasting from sunrise to sunset during Ramadan or the ninth month in the Islam calendar. Christians and Buddhists have similar mandates.

When we are sick, we instinctively fast. The same is true for animals. The point is fasting is natural. Fasting is an old concept that has been in practice for thousands of years. Fasting is far more natural than having six small meals throughout the day or eating every four hours.

The human body is quite equipped for fasting. Our bodies can certainly manage to function even on extended periods of skipping at least one meal in a day. Our hunter-gatherer ancestors were able to go to work and manage to make a kill after hours and hours of stalking their next meal. We can certainly manage too!

You probably get the idea behind intermittent fasting by now. But what's in it for you? In the next chapter, we lay out the best reasons why intermittent fasting can do you more good than harm.

Chapter 2

The Powerful Benefits of Intermittent Fasting

There's nothing overly complicated about Intermittent Fasting. It is simply an eating pattern. It is an alternating cycle of feasting and fasting. You divide the periods between when you're eating and fasting.

IF has been gaining notoriety in the weight loss arena. Aside from its weight loss benefits however, there's more to Intermittent Fasting than meets the eyes. There have been quite a number of research studies suggesting its powerful benefits it offers for the body and the brain. Among those health benefits include the following.

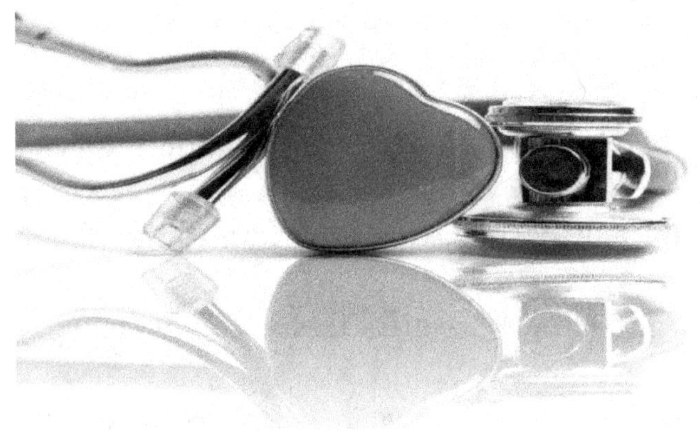

IF helps you take care of your health.

URL Source:

https://www.pexels.com/photo/bright-cardiac-cardiology-care-433267/

Intermittent Fasting leads to positive changes in the body.

Everyone's aware of the benefits of eating but did you know that not eating for a while can also be beneficial? We're talking about cellular level changes. So what happens when you skip a meal and fast?

1. Insulin blood level - The first change that occurs involves the insulin levels. During fasting, insulin blood levels drop significantly. Why is this important? If you're trying to lose extra weight, this is exactly what you want to happen. It is because lower insulin blood level is equivalent to a more efficient fat burning process.

2. Growth hormone - Another change that occurs during fasting concerns the human growth hormone. You see growth hormone can elevate as much as five times more during fasting. What does this mean for you? A higher level of growth hormone is ideal for weight loss. That's because it helps further with not only fat burning but also muscle gain.

3. Cellular repair - During the fasting period, cellular repair processes are stimulated. The body becomes much more efficient in eliminating waste materials that may have accumulated in the cells.

4. Gene expression - The genes also benefit from fasting. Molecules and genes associated with

disease protection and prevention as well as life longevity go through beneficial changes.

Lose weight without too much restriction.

The downside with tradition weight loss methods is the calorie-restricted diet. Losing weight is indeed a challenge and it feels a little bit more insurmountable and stressful with a limited food option. Counting calories is not exactly something you can look forward to doing. Dieters are overwhelmed with feelings of deprivation.

When you limit yourself too much in portions and in food options, craving can even become much more uncontrollable. The weight that may have lost in the process is much easier to regain. According to research, this is one of the top reasons why people abandon their diet halfway through before even getting results.

Intermittent fasting on the other hand, offers much more flexibility. With IF, you don't have to bother about dieting every single day of the week. After some time of restricting your calorie intake, it's easy to lose motivation. Because the IF method is about scheduling eating and fasting, it depends on time.

You have to follow the rules but it doesn't involve counting calories. This makes this method ideal for people who likes the idea of following rules rather than limiting their calorie intake. You don't have to eat less but you should not eat after a certain time. The schedule is up to you to design. This among other things make Intermittent Fasting an effective method for losing weight. It is neither too complicated nor too restricting to follow.

IF can help you lose belly fat.

Belly fat is the easiest to gain but the hardest to lose. Intermittent fasting can help you reach this goal. Although there are many health benefits to IF, most people who consider this regimen do so with the objective to lose weight in mind. With IF, you are encouraged to take fewer meals. This means you take fewer calories in the process provided that you do not compensate on your portions during your feasting period.

In addition to consuming fewer calories without the laborious task of counting, IF also works in enhancing your hormone function that plays a role in facilitating the process of weight loss. Intermittent fasting further promotes body fat breakdown to be used for energy. This is a result of reducing lower insulin levels and increasing growth hormone levels. Furthermore, IF can increase metabolic rate by as much as 3.6 or up to 14 percent. This means your body becomes much more efficient in burning calories.

For all these reasons, IF is an effective weight loss method because it works in two amazing ways. One, it helps decrease your calorie intake. Two, it helps burn more calories by firing up your metabolic rate.

A 2014 review backs up these claims. According to the researchers, the participants lost 3 to 8 percent of their initial weight in a course of 3 to 24 weeks. The participants also shed belly fat recording a 4 to 7 percent loss in their waist circumference. And for those who want to shed some weight but worry about muscle loss, IF is a far better option than a calorie restricted diet. That's because continuous calorie restriction can cause muscle loss, IF doesn't. Overall, this makes IF a great weight loss tool.

Intermittent Fasting works better for the long run.

Other weight loss diets challenge you to incorporate their method to your lifestyle permanently. It is easier said than done. The more likely scenario is losing the weight too fast and gaining it back eventually. With IF, the weight loss rate may be slower but you have a better chance of maintaining it. The simplicity of the method and the sacrifice-reward system is much easier to stick to in the long run.

Oxidative stress and inflammation can be reduced with IF.

Free radicals are unstable molecules that cause oxidative stress. These unstable molecules cause damage to important molecules. Oxidative stress can lead to premature aging. When not attended to properly, it can also lead to various chronic diseases.

There have been several studies that found how IF can help in enhancing resistance to oxidative stress. Moreover, it can help in fighting off inflammation.

Stimulate cellular repair processes with IF.

During fasting, the cells trigger a metabolic pathway referred to as autophagy. It involves waste removal at a cellular level. The cells break down and metabolize dysfunctional and broken proteins that accumulate within the cells over time. With an elevated autophagy, the body receives protection against various diseases which includes cancer and Alzheimer's.

IF may decrease the risk to diabetes.

Diabetes is among the top common diseases to date. In addition to people who are already suffering from the disease, the number of people with pre-diabetes is also on the rise. Diabetes is characterized by elevated blood sugar levels as a result of insulin resistance. To counteract diabetes or to prevent it at the very least, the aim is to reduce insulin resistance in order to decrease blood sugar levels.

According to the record of the United States Centers for Disease Control and Prevention or CDC, there are around 84.1 million individuals in the U.S. who have pre-diabetes. If the condition is not treated, it is more likely to develop to type 2 diabetes in the next 5 years.

How can we prevent pre-diabetes from developing to type 2 diabetes? A properly maintained weight, exercise and a healthy diet can all help. CDC explains as an individual loses weight, he/ she becomes more insulin-sensitive. It simply means blood sugar level remains low. As we eat, our bodies release insulin which goes to the bloodstream providing a steady supply of energy to the cells.

However, those with pre-diabetes are insulin-resistant. That means their blood sugar levels are always high.

More than any weight loss method, Intermittent Fasting can effectively help with reducing the risk to diabetes. That's because with IF, the body is required to produce insulin much less often. Remember, IF involves fasting and feasting. This is especially helpful to those with family history of diabetes or those who are already pre-diabetic.

There have been research studies supporting this claim. Researchers have found that a diet that mimics the fasting cycles could actually help in restoring insulin secretion and at the same time, aid in generating new pancreatic beta cells that are insulin-producing. The results in mice samples are quite promising. As a matter of fact, there have been early studies involving human cell samples and the results suggest a similar potential.

In human studies on IF, fasting blood sugar showed a reduction of 3 to 6 percent. On the other hand, fasting insulin recorded a decrease of 20 to 31 percent. In addition, mice studies found that IF may also help protect the kidneys from damage which is among the most severe complications diabetic people suffer from.

In other words, following an IF regimen can help protect individuals who are at high risk to type 2 diabetes. It is important to note however, that the results vary between genders. While men in general, can benefit from IF in reducing insulin resistance and lowering blood sugar levels as a result, women in general, may not enjoy the same benefits. There had been only one study to point out the difference, further research may be necessary.

IF can help keep your circadian rhythm in sync and prevent metabolic diseases at the same time.

The circadian rhythm is the body clock or the sleep/wake cycle. The National Sleep Foundation says it is a natural internal system that regulates the feelings of wakefulness and sleepiness in the course of a 24-hour period. What does this have to do with IF or dieting for that matter?

The body's sensitivity to insulin is elevated during the day. On the other hand, insulin sensitivity is lower at night. Again, this has to do with digestion. Researchers suggest that eating during nighttime may actually work against the body clock. In addition, there are certain foods that are taken before bed which are associated with weight gain as well as sleep disturbances. This is especially true when those foods are known to cause acid reflux. This is why eating before 6pm for instance, may actually do our bodies some good.

There is another research study suggesting that fasting may be able to cause a reset in the circadian clock. Sleeping at the right time can help restore the body. To respect our body clocks, we need to go to bed to sleep and rest. This way, we allow our bodies enough time to restore itself.

IF may help reduce the risk to cardiovascular diseases.

Heart disease is the biggest killer in the world. It causes around 610,000 deaths in the U.S. every year according the CDC. The best ways to prevent heart diseases is to lead a healthy lifestyle which means not smoking, limiting the consumption of alcohol, exercising and eating right. According to research, intermittent fasting may also help.

There are health markers linked to the risk of developing heart disease. Such health markers include blood sugar levels, inflammatory markers, blood triglycerides, LDL cholesterol and blood pressure among others. IF proves to address such risk factors.

There was one study that made participants follow an alternate-day fasting. The regimen was able to cause weight loss. At the same time, the participants showed a decrease in their total cholesterol and LDL cholesterol levels. They also recorded a reduction in triacylglycerol concentration and blood pressure. Researches emphasize that fasting does not necessarily mean starving. It simply means eating lesser.

Intermittent Fasting presents a formidable alternative to calorie restricted weight loss diets. In this method, you only restrict a couple of times a week instead of everyday. Because you eat fewer times, you get to reduce your calorie intake without thinking much about it.

Reduce your risk to Cancer through Intermittent Fasting.

Cancer is one of the scariest, most terrible diseases. There have been many speculations on how to prevent it. And fasting is one of them. The positive changes on metabolism caused by IF can be beneficial in the prevention of cancer. So far, studies have been limited to animals but the findings are promising. Some evidences have also been found on how fasting can help alleviate chemotherapy side effects in cancer patients.

Intermittent Fasting promotes brain health.

IF is not only good for the body, it also offers many benefits for the brain. Metabolic features affect the health of the brain. By reducing blood sugar and insulin levels, inflammation and oxidative stress, IF can also be beneficial for brain health. Intermittent fasting may also have a direct effect on brain function. A study in mice show how it helps in stimulating growth of nerve cells. Research also shows how it can elevate brain-derived neurotrophic factor or BDNF which is a brain hormone. A deficiency in BDNF is associated with many brain problems including depression. According to animal studies, IF may also protect the brain from damage as a result of stroke.

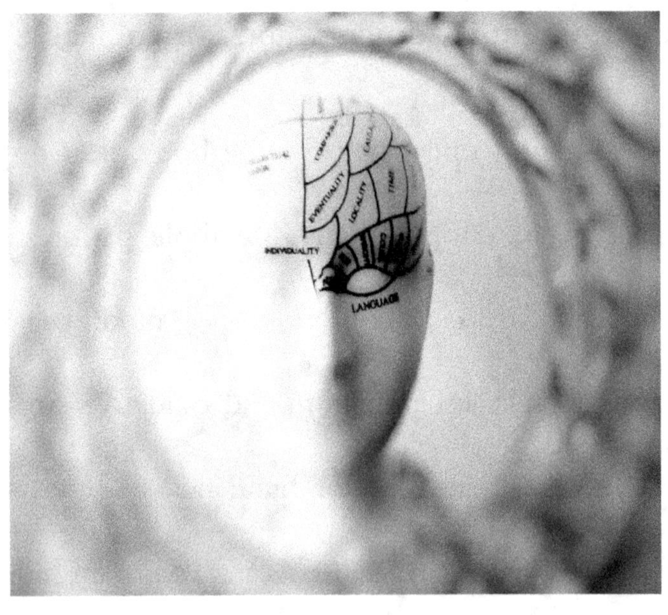

IF promotes brain health.

URL Source:

https://www.pexels.com/photo/photo-of-head-bust-print-artwork-724994/

Prevent neurodegenerative diseases with IF.

Alzheimer's disease is still the most widespread neurodegenerative disease in the world. Unfortunately, there is no cure for it. Prevention is critical and IF may just help in this cause.

A study in mice found that IF may help in delaying Alzheimer's onset. It also showed how IF can aid in reducing the severity of this neurodegenerative disease. In several case reports,

Alzheimer's symptoms were improved in 9 of 10 patients after a lifestyle intervention which included short-term fasts on a daily basis.

In addition to Alzheimer's, there have also been animal studies suggesting that IF may be able to provide a protective blanket against other neurodegenerative diseases such as Huntington's and Parkinson's disease. Hopefully, more human studies will be conducted to shed light to these findings.

Intermittent fasting may help you live longer.

A study found that fasting stimulates adaptive cellular stress responses. In other words, it helps the body manage stress better. It also helps in counteracting diseases.

Low-calorie diets have anti-aging benefits according to experts. In place of restrictive diets, intermittent fasting has the same effect. While you are not counting calories or limiting yourself too much, you consume fewer calories because of fasting.

Studies in mice showed that fasting can extend lifespan. The one group of mice that went through fasting every other day extended their lifespan by 83 percent compared to the group that did not fast. It is yet to be proven true for humans as well. The fact however, that intermittent fasting prompts the body to go through positive changes and prevent diseases may be enough evidence to prove how it can help us live a little longer by living a healthier life.

Who can benefit from Intermittent fasting?

Like all weight loss diets, intermittent fasting serves certain people best. An overweight person can benefit greatly from it. If you have reached a weight loss plateau, IF is an excellent way to jumpstart your metabolism. It can further boost your weight loss progress.

Even people with digestive problems can benefit from IF. If you have a sluggish digestion or experience digestive problems in the evening, you can have your supper at an earlier time and fast overnight.

It will help you not only lose weight but also ease your digestive issues.

Even if you think your body is in perfect shape and form, you can probably use some of these benefits from intermittent fasting. So, if you care about your overall health, let's get into the nitty gritty of IF in the succeeding chapters.

Chapter 3

How does Intermittent Fasting work?

When you skip a meal, you are eating less than you normally do on average. Minus one meal then that is equivalent to two meals rather than three. That's how you lose weight. By choosing to forego one meal a day, you are taking in a fewer number of calories in a given week. This will still be true even if you upgrade the two meals you have left in the day. Your overall consumption of calories will still be lesser than what you're used to.

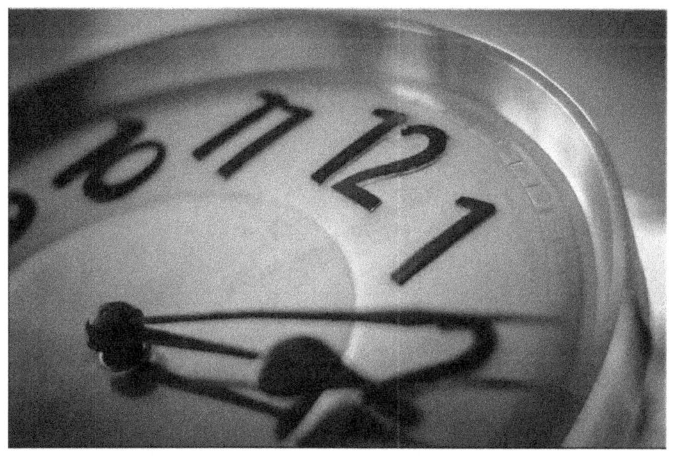

Intermittent fasting is about timing your meals.

URL Source:

https://www.pexels.com/photo/clock-close-up-time-280253/

There is one JAMA study that compared the results of intermittent fasting to calorie restricted diets. Those that fasted lost the same amount of weight as those that went through calorie restricted diets over one year. It makes sense, right? But there's more to intermittent fasting than this.

You probably know for a fact that foods are not created equal and so are calories. The timing or scheduling of your meals also affect the body and how it responds. This is why counting calories alone may not be enough.

Feasting versus Fasting

There are various ways that intermittent fasting can work. One of which is the difference between fasting and feasting. The human body operates differently during the period of fasting and the period of feasting.

Just like we favor some foods over others, the body also plays favorites. When we eat a mix of foods, the body burns sugar and carbohydrates first to convert to energy. That's because compared to any other energy food source, carbohydrates and sugar are readily convertible to energy. What is not burned and converted is stored as fat.

There is no first in first out rule. Whenever we eat, our body needs a few hours to process what we just consumed. It will try to burn as much as it can from what we just ate. The food we just consumed is readily available and much easier to burn. This is why it makes sense for our bodies to choose to process it as energy instead of burning stored fat.

What happens to the stored fat in our bodies then? When do their get their turn? As long as we are eating something new, the body will prefer to burn that. However, during the period of fasting when we let hours pass by without consuming anything, our bodies will be left without a choice but to withdraw from the fat it has been storing for energy. Without a recently consumed food to be burned as energy, the body looks into the next readily available energy source which is stored fat. This is exactly what we want to happen if our objective is to lose weight.

You may not like this next idea but it will absolutely help you lose more weight. To boost your burn, you may want to consider working out during your period of fasting. When you fast, your glycogen and glucose supply becomes depleted. This will help ensure more fat burning especially when you skip a pre-workout meal. In this case, the body becomes forced to take from the only energy source left. That is the stored fat in the cells.

Why Intermittent Fasting works?

The short answer to this question is insulin production and sensitivity. Every time you eat a meal, your body responds by producing insulin. If your body is sensitive to insulin, then your food consumption will be used as energy efficiently. During fasting, the body's sensitivity is elevated. In other words, when you are on a fasting period, your body goes through positive changes as far as insulin production and insulin sensitivity are concerned. Because of such changes, you are more likely to lose weight and build muscles.

Glycogen is "a substance deposited in bodily tissues as a store of carbohydrates. It is stored in the liver and the muscles. Like the food we consume, this starch can also be burned when the body finds it necessary. Now the body's glycogen level becomes depleted when we sleep which is a period of fasting (unless you sleepwalk your way to the kitchen to sleep eat). The glycogen level further decreases and burned when you work out. This way, a period of fasting combined with a period of training can further boost insulin sensitivity. So a meal taken after training becomes stored in a more efficient manner.

When you fast, workout and eat, the food will be converted to glycogen. It may be stored in the muscles or burned for energy in order to help with the body's recovery process. In this case, food stored as fat is at a minimum.

So what difference does it make to fast? On an average day without intermittent fasting, your sensitivity to insulin is at a normal level. Whatever food you consume will be stored as glycogen. Because there are sufficient glucose flowing in your bloodstream, the excess is likely to be stored as fat.

During a period of fasting, the growth hormone level is also elevated. This increase in the secretion of growth hormone, along with the decreased production of insulin and consequently, an increase in sensitivity to insulin all work together to prepare the body for fat loss and muscle growth. In simpler terms, through intermittent fasting, you can teach your own body the following things:

- To utilize what you eat more efficiently

- To burn fat for energy as you diminish your intake of new calories

More than losing weight, intermittent fasting can be used to promote muscle building as long as it is done properly.

Fed State versus Fasted State

In a fed state, the body is in the process of digesting food and absorbing it. This begins as you eat and it will last for about three or up to five hours when your body starts digesting and absorbing what you just consumed. In this state, the body finds it difficult to burn fat because one, the insulin levels are quite high and two, the body pulls energy from the most recently consumed meal.

The next state is the post-absorptive phase. In this state, the body is neither digesting nor absorbing food. It can last from eight or up to twelve hours counting after the last meal. This post-absorptive state leads to the fasted state when your body finds it easier to burn fat because one, the insulin levels are lower and two, the body is deprived of new calories to pull from for energy.

During a period of fasting, the body is ready to burn the fat which was not accessible in the fed state. The thing is, the body doesn't go to a fasted state until you have reached 12 hours after the last consumed meal. In other words, people rarely enter the fat burning state. It is when we intentionally skip a meal and follow intermittent fasting that we reach the fasted state also known as the fat burning state.

This is among the top reasons why a lot of individuals who get started on IF lose fat even if they don't change what they eat or their portions and without exercise. It is simply because fasting leads the body to the fat burning phase which is rarely entered in a normal meal schedule.

Chapter 4
Diet versus No-Diet Diet

You must be asking yourself this. If intermittent fasting can really deliver weight loss results, why have you heard of or read about it just now? And why do other diets recommend a meal plan and this one doesn't?

The simple answer is that the weight loss world has been told too many times about the "right" way of dieting, it gradually became the bible of losing weight. It is understandable to be doubtful when you start hearing of or reading about something new.

So let's talk about the most popular weight loss diet in the arena, the one that recommends six small meals a day. Let's study the reasons behind this diet, why it may work and why you have a better chance with intermittent fasting.

Consuming six small meals in a day may work because of the following reasons.

-It makes your body constantly burn extra calories.

-It can prevent overeating.

Six small meals a day can get your metabolism fired up.

In order to process the food that we eat, the body needs to burn some extra calories. One of the flagship theories of this diet is that the body will be forced to burn extra calories all day long as you consume small meals a day. The metabolism is fired up and works at an optimum capacity.

In principle, this argument sounds assuring. In reality however, there is a different story. The truth is there is not much difference between consuming 2000 calories throughout the day and taking the same amount in one seating. The body needs the same amount of energy and is more likely to burn similar amount of calories to process 2000 calories whether it is distributed in six small meals or taken in one big meal. In other words, you won't be burning more extra calories by consuming six small meals in a day.

Six small meals throughout the day can help prevent you from overeating.

Keeping yourself full throughout the day by eating small meals seems much better than starving yourself. If you have a problem controlling how much you eat, this may work. And if it is a real struggle, you may find it even more challenging to control your portions every time you snack. Because we're talking about small meals here, it is less likely for someone who struggles with portion control to feel full.

The simple truth is that although a six small meals a day plan may seem like the best fit for weight loss is likely not suitable for everybody. If you thrive on routine, this will probably work. On the other hand, it is more likely an impractical choice for many. Not everyone simply has the time to prep and pack six small meals for each day. After all, this diet plan requires small, measured, balanced and home-cooked meals.

Think of the cavemen days. They did not have to eat six small meals in equal portions throughout the day. Can you imagine how much of a trouble that could have been for them? They stayed lean and mean though. They would eat when they can. They fasted when necessary. They survived. Their bodies adapted well to those conditions and they functioned optimally.

With this said, intermittent fasting is far from perfect. It certainly isn't for everybody. This however, does not take away from the fact that...

-Intermittent fasting could work for your weight loss goals.

-IF makes losing weight much simpler.

-Intermittent fasting does not require a lot of time and money.

Intermittent fasting could work for your weight loss goals.

Restricting calorie intake does play a significant role in an effort to lose weight. Aside from counting calories and downsizing meals, fasting is another approach to calorie restriction. By skipping just one meal a day, you can significantly cut back on your calorie intake in the course of a week. Think about how much it would be in a month or in a year. In this sense, fasting can ensure consistent weight loss. It can also mean easier maintenance of weight.

IF makes losing weight much simpler.

Why would you complicate your life when there is a much simpler way to do things? With intermittent fasting, you don't have to worry about preparing, packing, eating and scheduling your small meals. The only thing you have to decide is your eating period. There are no special meals or recipes you have to learn to cook. There is no measuring of portions required.

Intermittent fasting does not require a lot of time and money.

One of the top reasons why a lot of people who start diets usually end up abandoning it is that they are overwhelmed about how much time, effort and money those diets require from them. Planning a weekly menu for three meals a day already takes up a lot of time, how much more would six meals a day require? It is not just about the time and effort. It is about the money too. Not everyone can afford a major overhaul in their eating lifestyle. With intermittent fasting however, you don't have to

concern yourself about such things. In principle, you

are saving yourself time and money by eating two

instead of three time a day!

Chapter 5
Choose Your Fasting Schedule!

Another great thing about intermittent fasting is that there are various options for it. You can choose a schedule that will be the easiest to integrate into your lifestyle. There are a total of five intermittent fasting protocols. Your choice should coincide with your current lifestyle and your planned level of training. The most commonly used are these three.

- Daily Intermittent Fasting or the 16:8

- Weekly Intermittent Fasting or the EAT STOP EAT Protocol

- Alternate Day Fasting

Daily Intermittent Fasting or 16:8

This is the Lean Gains method and probably the most popular among all the protocols. That's because it is the easiest to adapt. It causes very little disruption and with that, it is the easiest to stick to.

In this protocol, you ought to assign a 16 hour fasting period and an 8 hour feeding period. It doesn't matter what time you start or stop as long as you fit it in your daily schedule. For instance, you wake up at 6:00 am, have lunch at 12 noon, dinner at 7:00pm and go to bed at 9:00pm. In this regular schedule, your period of eating starts at 6:00 am and ends at 7:00 pm. That's a 13-hour window. If you are to adapt 16:8 intermittent fasting, you have to reduce the feeding period to an 8-hour window. The easiest way to do this is to skip breakfast, eat lunch like you usually do at 12 noon and maybe stick to dinner at 7:00 or move it to 8:00 pm.

You should pick a window that works well with your schedule. The key here is to make it as simple as possible. Usually though, it is easiest to skip the meal that you typically have on your own. If you are used to having breakfast alone, maybe skip that and join your family and friends for lunch and dinner.

It is easier to turn something into a habit when you are doing it every day. This intermittent fasting protocol is flexible enough allowing you to easily do it. You don't have to think about it constantly. You can stick to your regular schedule, only you have to teach yourself to eat only at certain times. And by cutting one meal a day, you end up burning fat and losing weight.

If you can commit to this daily schedule every single time, 100 percent, you will probably reach your weight loss goals in no time. Some people can only commit to it 90 percent of the time and allow themselves to do whatever they feel like on the remaining 10 percent. It is not a mortal sin to do this as long as you keep your 90 percent commitment.

For instance, there are rare incidents when you may run to a friend you haven't seen for a while, invites you for a snack at 10:am on a Sunday, you can go for it. In this case, you can probably adjust your feeding schedule from 10:00 am to 6:00 pm for that day. Or count it as 10 percent and proceed to your schedule as usual.

Here is a sample Daily Intermittent Fasting schedule:

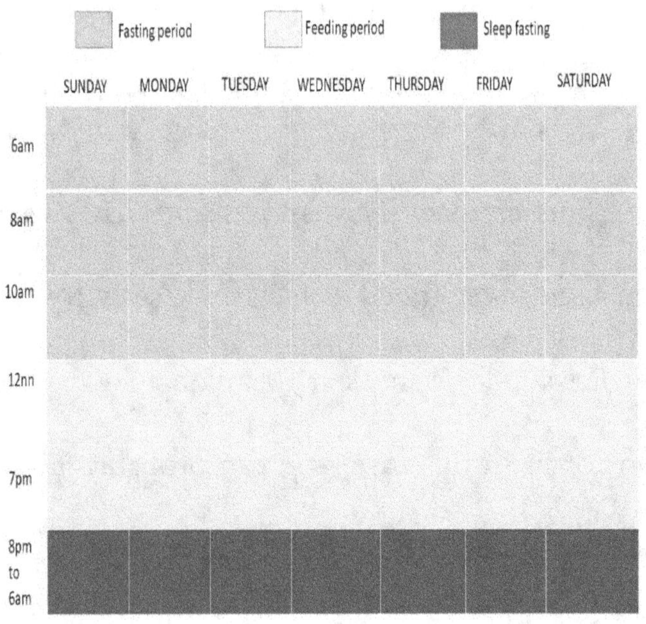

Who is most likely to succeed in this protocol?

If you are not a morning person who usually doesn't have time to cook breakfast anyway, it will be easier to skip the meal. You can have coffee as long as you skip the bagel. Or if you usually come home late, too tired to cook dinner, you might as well skip it. In this case, skipping either of the meals will help you stick to your 8 hour feeding period.

The daily intermittent fasting protocol is also suited for you if you are someone who thrives on a schedule. If you are most comfortable in a routine, you are most likely to succeed in this IF method.

What is the best feeding period?

There is no recommendation as far as feeding period or window is concerned. The most important thing is the eating is reduced to 8 hours a day. However, the most commonly used is between 11:00 am to 7:00 pm. If this blends well with your current way of living, that's great! Otherwise, you are free to choose your own.

Does it really have to be every day?

The recommendation is for you to follow the 16:8 protocol 7 days a week. The beginning is the most challenging just because we are all used to eating at certain times of the day. There is an adjustment period to every new habit you are trying to build so just give it sometime and you will get used to it. The goal at the start is to build the habit and overcome the urge to eat according to the clock. If you are to make it a habit, it is best to do the 16:8 fasting every single day. You have to be consistent about it until it becomes the new norm!

Let's say you think you can stick to this protocol from Sunday to Friday but will likely deviate on Saturdays, is that allowed? There are no intermittent fasting police as of yet and you're free to do whatever you like. But to avoid getting frustrated or feeling guilty about it, you must make this declaration before getting started.

Remember the 90 percent commitment I mentioned earlier? It's alright to break the rules 10 percent of the time. Of course, it is not ideal BUT if you think that is the best you can do, no one's going to crucify you!

Weekly Intermittent Fasting or the EAT STOP EAT Protocol

Occasional fasting also has its benefits. The weekly fasting protocol is usually applied by those who wants to give intermittent fasting a try out. Here is a sample schedule.

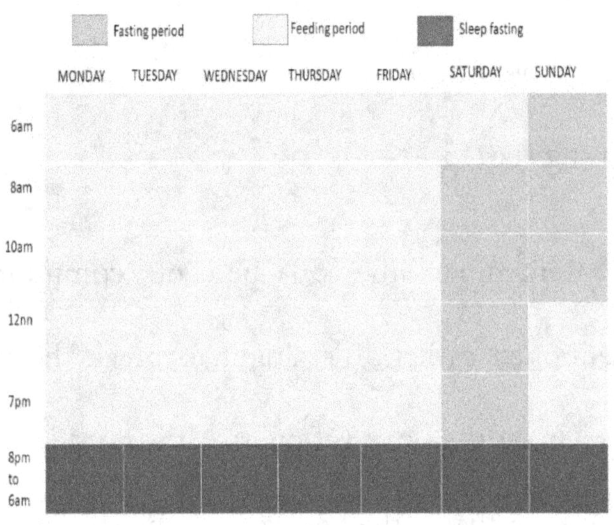

In this example, you go about you schedule from Monday to Friday as usual. Breakfast is taken on

Saturday morning at 6:00am. Fasting starts after that. The next meal taken should be Sunday lunch.

If your goal is to lose weight, this protocol may do very little for that goal. However, this is a great option for after the holidays. It allows your body to cleanse. And there are plenty of ways to do it. Although it may not be the greatest for losing weight, it does have health benefits of cleansing.

Basically, you're choosing one or two days in the week to do the fasting at your most convenient time. The main objective here is not to maximize weight loss but to simply realize that there is no need to consume food all the time.

The biggest challenge you have to face here is getting past the mental conditioning that skipping meals is bad. This is especially true if you have never broken the eating "rules" before. When you get past your first 20 to 24 hours of fasting, it will be an enlightening experience. You won't die if you skip meals all day. The world will not end. I bet my life on it!

Who is best suited to follow this protocol?

This is a great option if you are the type who likes eating breakfast and simply cannot let it go. It allows you to be a king in the morning in most days of the week. It is also suited for you if you travel quite often. Some find a longer fast more advantageous on a trip.

Or if there are times when you simply are too busy for food.

When is the best fasting time?

The best fasting time depends on your own schedule. Some people may prefer to do it on a weekend simply because their Saturday and Sunday schedules are more flexible for fasting. In general, however, busy days may be more suitable for fasting. It may sound crazy for you at first because you're thinking, busy days are when you need to have your full energy, hence, a meal is a must. Let me ask you though, on your busiest day, do you really enjoy meals or you just force yourself to eat because it's "time" for a meal?

Fasting works well on busy days for two major reasons. One, time flies when you have too much to think about and too much to do. On the other hand, idle times create boredom and you are likely to feel the urge to fill that boredom with a chow down! Two, it's actually good for productivity. Remember, your body has deposits that can be used for energy so you don't have to worry about fainting while working. If you're afraid of losing focus, drink some water. When you need a break, have some tea. It's better than choking on a sandwich you are less likely to finish anyway!

In any case, you can choose a day or days of the week for fasting. And on these fasting days, make it your goal to skip meals between 20- and 24-hour periods. This includes your fasting time during sleep which accounts for about 7 to 10 hours.

Is it okay to do fasting more than twice a week?

For this protocol, one day in a week fasting for 20 to 24 hours is best. You probably can increase it to 2 days but it is not recommended to go beyond fasting for 40 to 48 hours straight. If you want to lose weight, there are other healthy ways to do it. Consider trying other intermittent fasting protocols that can help you meet your goals. It is important to find a good balance. In the case of longer fasting, it is still important to make sure you are consuming enough calories on the days you are not fasting.

Alternate Day Fasting

The rules of this protocol are pretty simple. Basically, you follow the 16:8 protocol on alternate days. If you skipped breakfast on Sunday, take it on Monday, fast again on Tuesday and resume regular schedule on Wednesday, etc.

Below is a sample schedule:

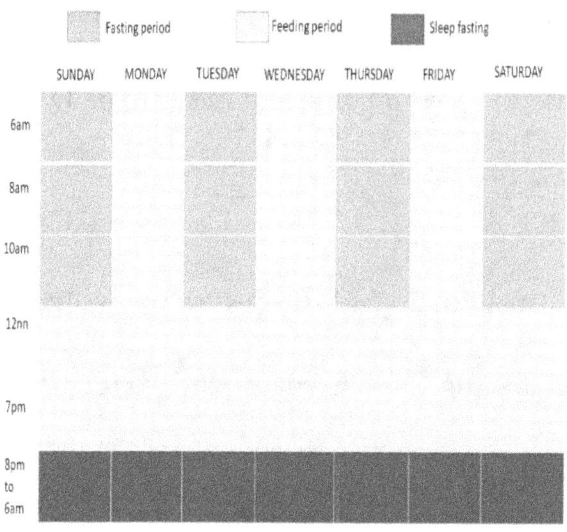

So you might be thinking if this will actually work? Technically, you're still cutting back on calories by skipping breakfast four times a week. Your body still goes through a fasting phase and fat burning state every other day so following this protocol can still lead to weight loss. It is best suited for you if you are hesitant about letting go of your kingly status at breakfast. It can also be a stepping stone for when you decide to up your game and move to daily intermittent fasting.

An alternative to this protocol involves a 20 to 24 hour fasting on alternate days. Here is a sample schedule.

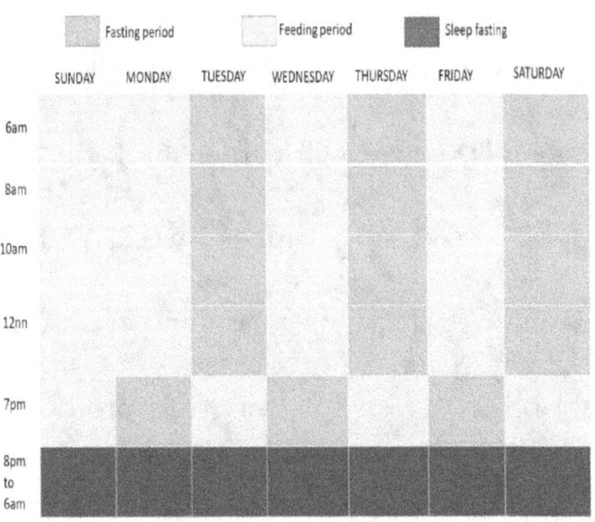

In this example, you skip dinner on Monday and the next meal you're going to have is dinner on Tuesday. You have breakfast and lunch on Wednesday but skip dinner. You won't have breakfast and lunch on Thursday but have dinner, etc.

This protocol allows you to have longer fasting periods consistently while making sure you consume at least one meal every single day. In principle, this protocol can lead to increase IF benefits. It is usually used in research studies but as far as real world application, it is not that popular.

It is probably much better than fasting 20-24 hours for more than two days straight. It will definitely boost weight loss results if you feel you have a lot to shed but for a beginner, this protocol may demand too much from you. It is definitely something to think about.

Chapter 6
Other Fasting Schedule Options

In addition to those mentioned in the previous chapter, there are other intermittent fasting protocols to choose from. Such options include the following.

- TT Fasting Protocol

- The 5:2 Protocol

- The Warrior Protocol

Remember, intermittent fasting is not a one-size-fits-all no-diet diet. The protocols are in place to give you options so you can choose which one best fits your goals and your current lifestyle.

TT Fasting Protocol

Among the intermittent fasting protocols, this is probably the easiest to follow. Remember that the fat burning state is achieved 12 hours after your last meal. In this case, you don't really have to skip a meal. Fasting occurs while you are sleeping. You just have to make sure to have a 12-hour difference between dinner and breakfast.

For instance, you usually wake up at 6:00 am and have your breakfast by 7:00 am. You will then have to consume your last meal of the day at 7:00 pm. Wait to complete your 12-hour window until you start breaking your fast.

For this protocol, a few things have to be emphasized. First, it is recommended that you veer away from having small snacks throughout the day. Second, you should focus instead on having three full meals. Third, this may not maximize your weight loss results but it will still allow you to shed some. The results may be minimal but it is a good start.

Who is most suited for the TT protocol?

If you are quite the nervous kind and you are still hesitant about fasting, this protocol is a gentle start. It gives you a chance to ease into intermittent fasting until you figure out if it is right for you. If you still have reservations about committing to a daily intermittent fasting but do recognize the benefits and positive changes it can contribute to your life, this makes a good choice. This protocol is also suited for people who struggle with late night cravings. It is an excellent way to curb those urges because it is simple to do and easy to follow.

When to have the 12-hour fast?

The natural choice is in the evening while you sleep. When you're sleeping and dreaming, you don't have to worry about getting hungry. A lot of people are more comfortable too with fasting when they have no activities planned out other than rest and sleep.

The other option is to fast when you are busy. 12 hours is nothing when you have so much to do. Time flies when you have a lot of things on your mind and you're driving yourself crazy to productivity. At any given point, you may get headaches. Relax. You're not dying! It is the body's normal response to the change you're trying to make. The headaches can be eased by drinking plenty of water. Staying hydrated is recommended during fasting.

What to do when you're just too hungry?

Old habits are hard to break. If you're used to having little snacks from time to time, it can be especially challenging to stop all of a sudden. Your body is conditioned to eat at certain times of the day.

It's not real hunger. Be patient and focus on something else other than food and stay busy. When the hunger becomes too much to bear, you can always get yourself a glass of water. Instead of chowing down, you can have a cup of coffee or tea.

What does a regular breakfast look like to you?

Do you eat breakfast like a kid? Milk and cereals? Milk and anything starchy? If this is how your typical breakfast looks like, it has to go through some changes. Focus on protein instead and healthy fats. Vegetable omelet is a good idea. If you are to go for carbs, try complex carbohydrates.

Eat in a slow manner. Chew your food meal. Avoid making it a timed activity. Find a way to enjoy it.

Is training a good idea during fasting?

Training during fasting is perfectly alright. However, if you have not fasted before, it is best to allow your body to adjust to the new routine first. In the beginning, it may be best to break your fast before you resume your training. And when you do, ease into it slowly. You may have a more difficult time if you are used to snacking or eating as part of your pre-workout regimen.

The 5:2 Protocol

It's called 5:2 because in this protocol, you are to have 5 days of full calorie meals and 2 days consisting of lower calorie meals. In essence, you won't go a day without consuming new calories. There is no recommendation on which two days to have your lower calorie meals. The choice depends on what you're comfortable with.

At the mere mention of calorie, you can probably make a guess why this protocol is not very popular. That's because for two days, you will have to count calories and make sure you don't go over the mark.

Is the 5:2 Protocol suited for you?

If the amount of food you eat does not matter and you feel comfortable reducing your meal amount in some days, this can work for you. "Dieting" is most difficult to do when you are surrounded by people who bonds on meals. Now, if you like a regular meal schedule either because of your family life or simply a lifestyle choice, this protocol may be suitable. It is best if you can spare two days from your week to have lower calorie meals and if you can find it easy to integrate in your work and training schedule too.

What does the two low calorie days look like?

First of all, he low calorie days consists of 500 calories. In other words, for two days of the week, you are only to consume a 500 calorie meal a day. Some diets will recommend spreading the 500 calorie allowance throughout the day in little 100 calorie snacks. However, as we mentioned earlier, 100 calories won't be enough to keep you satisfied anyway. Intermittent fasting recommends that the 500 calorie meal target should be taken at once. In this case, choose when to have this meal: breakfast, lunch or dinner.

Is it recommended to have these two days on a weekend?

This protocol is not like the EAT STOP EAT protocol where you can fast two days straight. You can probably do so later on but in the beginning, it is best to space the two days out. Let's say you have your first day on Tuesday and your next second day on Friday. You're not stuck on your initial two-day choice for eternity. Change it up as you please. And as you get the hang of it, you can probably do the two days in a row.

What can I have for 500 calories?

500 calories in not just about portion control. You may be surprised at just how much you can get for 500 calories if you're making the right choice. A good example of a 500 calorie meal is protein with your preferred vegetables. Carbohydrates are high in calorie content. If you want to maximize the calorie allowance, it is best to go for protein that can keep you feeling full for longer.

Below is a sample schedule.

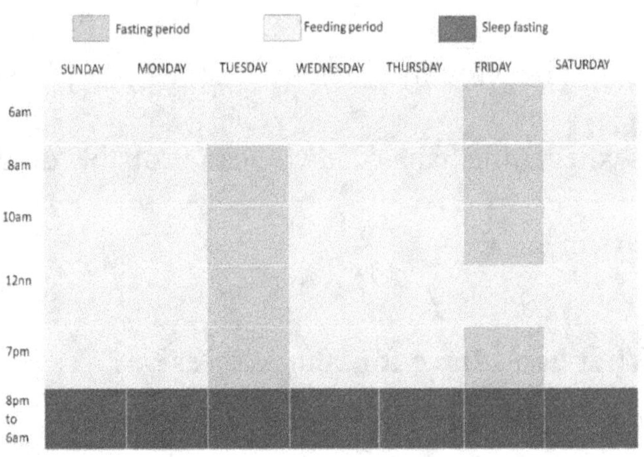

In this example, Tuesday and Friday are the low calorie days. On Tuesday, you take your 500 calorie allowance during breakfast. The following day and Thursday are regular meal days. On Friday, you save your 500 calorie meal for lunch. Your next meal is Saturday breakfast.

This is not written in stone. It is just an example to demonstrate how the protocol works. Feel free to choose your schedule

The Warrior Protocol

This protocol is not for the fainthearted. It is probably the most difficult of all the protocols. The warrior protocol requires 20 hours of fasting with only 4-hour period of eating. The recommendation is to schedule the feasting at dinner. You will not consume anything during the day. All your calories should be taken in the evening within a 4-hour window.

With this protocol, your daily schedule will look like this or something like it.

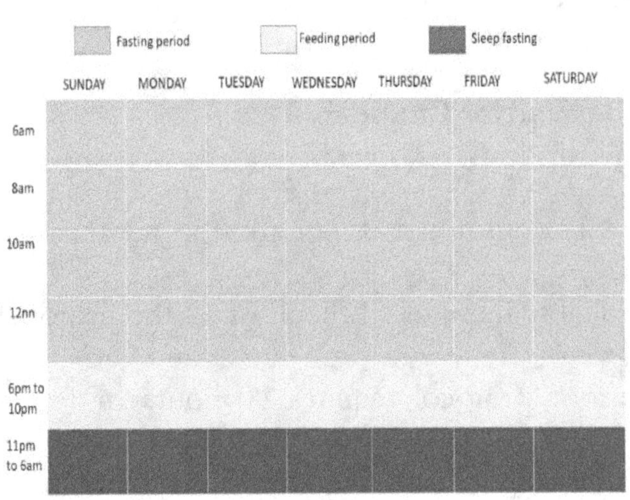

Is the Warrior Protocol suited for you?

This is on the extreme side of fasting and it is probably for you if you are the type that enjoys taking on a challenge. If you seem to always be busy with no time to spare for anything else other than work, the warrior protocol may be a piece of cake. If you're always occupied with a hundred important things, hunger is a piece of cake.

If you are used to not having breakfast, simply because you don't feel hungry when you wake up, this protocol will prove to be much simpler for you. If you have no interest in snacking and much less on preparing or packing food, fasting for 20 hours won't be a big deal. And if you tend to have more time in the evening to enjoy a meal, it will definitely work out. If one or more of these "if" scenarios apply to you, the warrior protocol may just be a great choice.

What is allowed during the 20-hour fasting window?

During the fasting period, you are allowed to have some water. Coffee and tea will do too. It is important to keep your fast until you reach the 4-hour feeding window. It is essential to keep hydrated while fasting. This will help curb the hunger and keep you healthy as well. Make sure you have enough water throughout the day.

Does this mean I can consume all my calories at dinner?

The warrior protocol essentially is about depriving yourself from anything other than water and non-caloric beverages until the 4-hour window comes then you feast! It's not just eating. It's literally feasting because in principle, you must consume all your calories for the day during this period.

Again, let's emphasize that not all calories are equal. This means you have to be a little picky about what you eat. Ideally, you should have whole foods. Your meal should be a balance of fats, carbs and proteins. Other intermittent fasters even have for themselves protein shakes as pre-bed snack. Cottage cheese, nuts and seeds are also ideal snack choices.

Is the IF Warrior Protocol meant to be done every day?

Just like the 16:8 daily intermittent fasting protocol, this one has to fit in to your daily schedule.

It will be challenging for the first few days or weeks.

Your body will eventually get accustomed to this eating system, you just have to give it time.

Chapter 7
Intermittent Fasting and Women

As it turns out, intermittent fasting affects women and men in different ways. Combined with physical training program, IF can help men build lean muscles. Depending on the protocol followed, weight loss can be achieved too while minimizing muscle loss. In addition to these physical changes, men can also enjoy the healing benefits of intermittent fasting such as disease prevention and longer, healthier life.

Let's be clear. Intermittent fasting is not for everyone. Although some report adverse side effects, others significantly benefit from it. It is safe to say that the effects of intermittent fasting vary depending on gender, individual disposition, and lifestyle and health status. However, in general, intermittent fasting can be followed safely. In fact, it can offer a long list of health benefits, help heal the body on a cellular level and extend life.

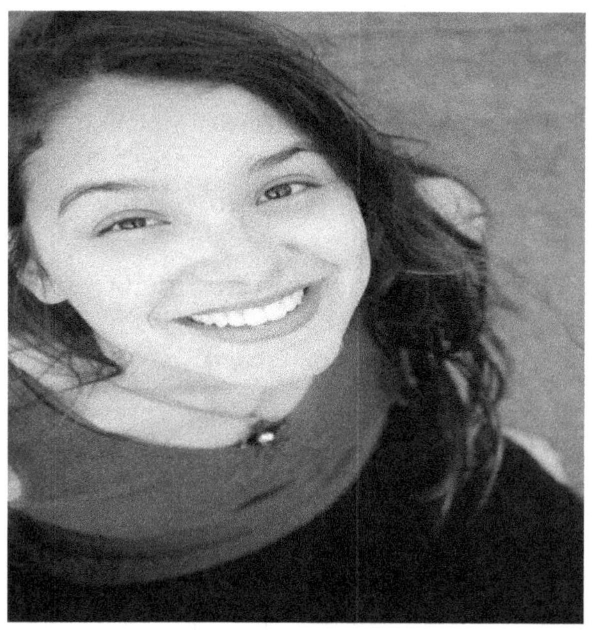

Intermittent fasting does not exactly have magical benefits on women?

URL Source:

https://www.pexels.com/photo/adolescent-adult-beautiful-brunette-312492/

So, how does it affect women?

In a study published on PubMed, researchers concluded that intermittent fasting can in fact, "be prescribed as a safe medical intervention as well as a lifestyle regimen which can improve women's health in many folds." Most of these studies however, focused on fasting in combination with calorie restriction. In order to extract a more conclusive evidence, further studies are required.

There is quite a number of smaller sample studies citing the varying effects of IF on genders. One study cited that while glucose response did not change in men and insulin response was significantly reduced, the results in women varied after completing a 3-week treatment. According to the study, insulin response did not change but glucose response became slightly impaired. The study involved 8 non-obese men and 8 non-obese women.

Another study was conducted on 8 women. Their menstrual cycle were evaluated after fasting for 72 hours. The researchers concluded that there were profound metabolic changes in the women but did not affect their menstrual cycle. The participants had normal menstrual cycles.

In a study involving 11 women, after fasting for 72 hours, the participants were reported to show the expected metabolic responses. However, they also recorded an increase in cortisol levels which is related to stress. Moreover, their central circadian clocks advanced as a result of fasting. This can possibly throw off normal sleeping patterns.

The studies cited above only worked with small sample sizes. They also used fasting methods different from those we discussed in the book. With all these noted, it can be concluded from these limited body of research that while fasting allows men to reap weight loss benefits in relation to insulin and glucose responses, women were affected negatively.

Who should definitely NOT attempt intermittent fasting?

Because the female body works differently, you have to be a little more cautious when trying out new changes in your routine. And if any of the following applies, you should best avoid intermittent fasting.

- You are with child.

- You have suffered from an eating disorder.

- You suffer from chronic stress.

- You have a sleeping problem.

- You have never tried any kind of diet.

- You have never attempted to exercise in your lifetime.

Until there is enough evidence with larger sample sizes and tackle the long-term effects of intermittent fasting on female subjects, it is probably in your best interest to stay out of it in the meantime.

The bottom line is we are all unique. Naturally, we are affected by IF, or any regimen for that matter, differently. If you are a woman reading this and considering to attempt intermittent fasting whether for the sole purpose of getting in shape or for other health benefits, you may want to pause the attempt and try other things instead.

Focus on the quality of your food.

Instead of fasting, you may want to try to evaluate your total calories. It is not about counting them. Rather, you should choose better quality of food. The quality stuff will give you more bang for your calorie count.

Get on a workout regimen.

If dieting doesn't work out for you to get in shape, you may perhaps want to try the other way. That is to work your body instead. It is not the most pleasant thing especially if you're not exactly the physical type of person but the effort could be worth it. Get off your comfort zone and exercise. Do it regularly!

Manage stress better.

Find ways to manage your stress levels. Stress is a bitch and it is known to cause various problems. If left unchecked, stress can even lead to diseases. And the simplest way of relieving stress is to make sure you get plenty of rest. Sleep well and sleep enough.

What if you still want to give it a shot?

You have been warned but your curiosity for intermittent fasting is getting the better of you. And you want to give it a shot anyway. As a grown woman, the choice is yours! It is your body after all and when it comes to your body, you should know best.

Do not try IF on a whim. I recommend that you speak to your doctor about it. Have yourself checked. If it requires blood work, so be it. You may just have a different response.

Get a clearance from your doctor first. Ideally, consult a professional who is knowledgeable in intermittent fasting and its protocols. And once you get a green light, monitor your results closely. Listen to your body carefully and respond accordingly.

Chapter 8

Frequently Asked Questions about IF

Let's set proper expectations first. You may have a hundred questions running on your mind right now. You're curious and excited but a little hesitant. We will address those questions in this chapter.

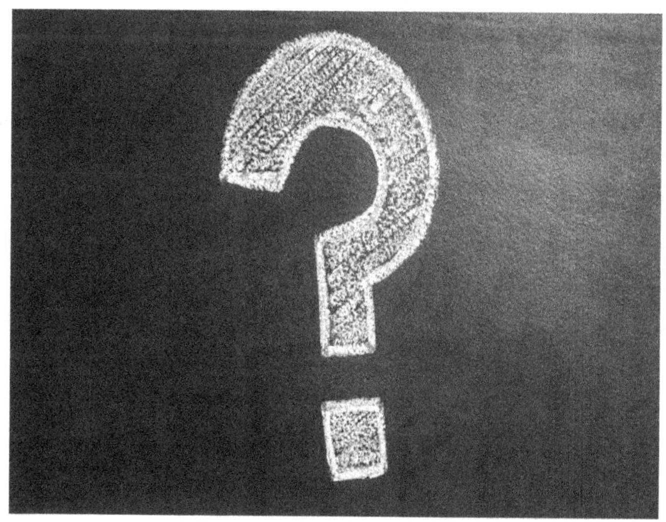

URL Source:

https://www.pexels.com/photo/ask-blackboard-

chalk-board-chalkboard-356079/

What are the side effects?

Let's talk about the biggest concerns a lot of

people have about intermittent fasting. Food gives us

joy and energy. When that is taken away, it is one hell

of an adjustment. People are hesitant of IF because they are afraid that without food, they will be miserable. It can ruin their day if they don't have breakfast. They may lose focus, energy and completely ineffective at work.

When you transition from having access to food all the time to following an intermittent fasting protocol, naturally, it can create a jolt to your life. It is the same for everyone. The transition period can last for a few days but you will be surprised how fast the body can adapt especially if you keep an open mind about it. It is quite natural to feel a bit lethargic and grumpy when you start skipping meals. This is just a result of your eating habits. When you're used to something and you try to break it, you will of course experience a little jolt. And that's just what it is.

Studies have proven that fasting does not adversely affect activity, cognitive performance, mood and sleep. One study reported such results after observing participants who have fasted for two days. The feelings of being out of focus are all in the mind. When you do experience some unpleasant side effects like feelings of hunger, you can always calm it down by drinking water.

Won't I get hungry?

Of course you will get hungry. At some point, you will really get hungry. However, it is important to understand that such feelings of hunger are created by the habits built into your system. The hunger struggle can be more pronounced when you have more excess weight. This will last as long as your body is adjusting. If you have the patience to endure, you will make it through the adjustment phase and you will get used to your new routine. Neither your physical nor your cognitive abilities are impaired due to fasting.

If I'm not eating, where do I obtain my energy?

Carbohydrates is a readily available source of energy. As explained in the previous chapters, you have stored energy in the form of fats. That's where your body can draw energy from.

Training on a fasted state is not only safe. As a matter of fact, it is ideal. According to research studies, when you train while your body is on a limited supply of carbohydrates, the muscle cells are stimulated. They will be able to adapt to the new condition and will begin facilitating the production of energy through fat oxidation. In simpler terms, the body on a fasted state can become more efficient with fat burning.

Although I like the idea of training during fasting, I have a regular work schedule. How do I make it work?

You have various options and such includes the following.

1. Adjust your feasting and fasting periods.

If you've chosen to do the 16:8 protocol, you can simply adjust your feeding and fasting schedule. Instead of skipping breakfast and having your feasting period from 11 am to 7 pm, you can set your feasting window after your training.

2. Have a small and big meal.

Another option is to stick to your feasting window between 11 am and 7 pm but have a smaller meal during lunch and pack up for post-workout. This is assuming you're doing your workout after 5pm onwards. Your small meal at lunch should be much more focused on protein and fats. Your big meal with carbs should be taken after your training.

3. Think about a protein supplement.

If you're on the 16:8 protocol and would rather workout before heading to work but skip breakfast, you may want to consider taking a protein supplement post workout. You can also wait until lunch but if your body doesn't respond well to this, you can always have the protein post workout supplement.

4. Consider another protocol.

You have other options as far as IF protocol is concerned. For instance, you can have alternate day fasting and workout on the days you're not skipping any meals.

Just remember that the rules of intermittent fasting are not written in stone. The beauty of this no-diet diet is in its flexibility. You can find multiple ways to make it work for you and fit it into your routine and lifestyle. The best thing to do is to avoid overthinking it, simply do what you can!

Won't I lose muscle because of fasting?

Not everyone aims to simply slim down. Some aims to have leaner muscles but this will not be possible if intermittent fasting can cause muscle loss. The good news is, it doesn't! We have been brainwashed by the supplement industry that our bodies require 30 grams of protein every couple of hours. Otherwise, our bodies will use the muscles instead, break it down and burn for energy. As it turns out, this is just a marketing ploy. There is no truth in this.

The fact is that the human body works excellently in preserving muscles. It continues to do so even when we are fasting. Also, the absorption of protein does not just take place over a few hours. It can in fact, take many hours. In other words, it does not matter whether we consume protein in shorter periods of time or on extended periods spread out throughout the day.

Can my body go on starvation mode?

Starvation mode is real and serious. However, for the body to go on starvation mode, it will take a much longer fast. Intermittent fasting only recommends 16 hours of fasting a day, 20-24 hours a day or 48 hours at the most and nothing longer. Before the body reaches starvation mode, it will require a much longer period of fasting. Needless to say, the recommendations of intermittent fasting are on the safe side.

How much am I allowed to eat on IF?

The answer here is quite simple. You should always eat according to your goals. If your objective is to lose weight, your daily calorie intake should be lesser than what you need. On the other hand, if you wish to bulk up, your daily calorie intake should be bigger than you can burn.

My suggestion is this. Eat your normal portions as you begin intermittent fasting. Monitor your weight. Track your performance. If you are achieving your goals with your normal-sized meals and you are content with your progress, there is no need to change anything. On the other hand, if you are not losing weight for instance, take it as a clue that you may be eating too much. Monitor your calorie intake for about a week. Aim for at least 10 percent reduction. Track your progress. If you're still not making any, you may need to reduce more. Do the reductions gradually. Apply reductions only when necessary.

Can everyone benefit from intermittent fasting?

In general, anyone can reap the amazing health benefits of IF. However, the experience may be a little more complicated for people who suffer from diabetes, hypoglycemia or have problems with blood sugar regulation. As a general rule, if you are suffering from any health condition and taking medications for it, you should always consult with your doctor first before trying anything new.

Chapter 9

Intermittent Fasting and Ketogenic Diet

So far, we have debunked a couple of myths. First is about how breakfast isn't really a necessity. Second was about how fasting can actually be good for your health and well-being. Third was about muscle building and so on. We certainly have room for more. So prepare yourself for another eye-opener. This time it's about the notion of fats. Guess what? Fats are actually good for you!

Intermittent fasting in itself, can produce great results. However, there is a diet that can work well with IF. It's called the Ketogenic Diet.

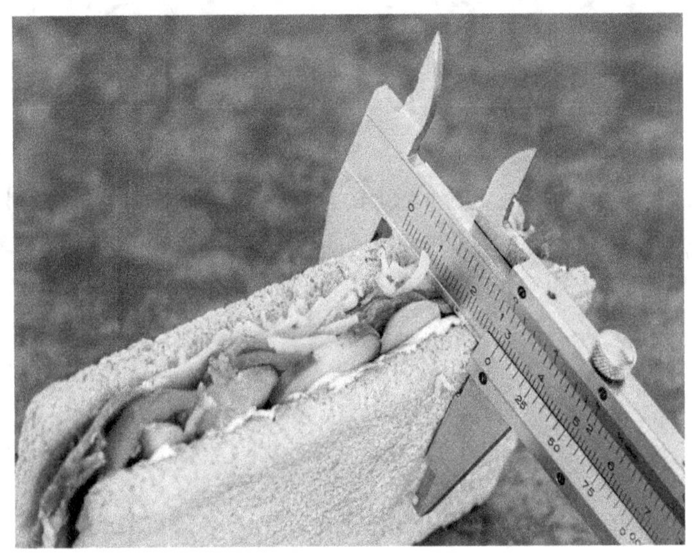

Measure your carbs!

URL Source:

https://www.pexels.com/photo/food-sandwich-eat-fitness-37417/

What is the Keto Diet?

Ketogenic is also known as the low carb diet or low carb high fat. That pretty sums up what this diet is all about. To elaborate, let me explain what happens in the body when we consume high carb meals like most of us do on a daily basis. When we eat foods that are rich in carbohydrates, our bodies produce glucose and insulin.

Glucose is the molecule that is easiest to convert to energy. In other words, it is readily available energy. Hence, it is the body's go-to energy source. To process glucose, the body produces insulin. Insulin is responsible for distributing energy derived from glucose throughout the body.

With glucose as the body's primary energy source, fats take a back seat. Our meals usually consist of carbohydrates, protein and fats. We now know that carbs are processed first, any excess is stored by the body. Clearly, it is not fats that make us fat. The real culprit is carbs!

If on the other hand, we lower our carb intake, the body will be forced to enter a state of ketosis. It is a metabolic state, a natural process where the body enters in order to survive in cases when the consumption of food is low. In the state of ketosis, the body produces ketones which is a product of fat breakdown in the liver.

To reach ketosis, we do not necessarily need to starve our bodies from calories. We only need to deprive it of carbohydrates. You will be amazed at how adaptive the human body is. When we lower or eliminate carbs from our diets and increase our intake of fats, our bodies will learn to burn fats and turn it into a primary source of energy. When we reach our optimal ketone levels, we can lose weight and we can even boost our physical and mental performance.

Benefits of a Ketogenic Diet

Like intermittent fasting, the ketogenic diet has faced many criticisms. But if you look closely into the science behind it, you will realize just how beneficial it is. Below are some of its top benefits.

1. It will help you lose weight.

Studies have proven that ketogenic diet can help you lose weight. By burning fat instead of carbs, you put your body into a fat burning state. Obviously, this will make you shed some unwanted weight. If you have tried a high-carb, low fat diet before, you will be delighted to know that keto diet can lead to better results, especially in the long run.

2. Keto will help you control your blood sugar level.

Low calorie diets have nothing on keto. Studies have reported that a ketogenic diet works more effectively in helping individuals control their blood sugar levels. It has been proven to help in managing and preventing diabetes. Pre-diabetic and Type II diabetes patients can benefit significantly from adapting a ketogenic diet. That's because keto focuses on the quality of foods you consume rather than counting your calorie intake.

3. It will help you improve your mental focus.

Carbs causes huge spikes in your blood sugar. This is actually bad for the brain. To function properly, the brain needs a steady source. Glucose gets burned fast. What happens is, your brain gets a jolt and then crashes.

A lower carb intake will help avoid these spikes. Ketones are actually an excellent fuel source for the brain. And it can help improve your ability to focus.

4. It can help increase your energy level.

If you need a sudden spike of energy, go for carbs! However, this is not good at all, all the time. To function more properly, the body needs a more reliable source of energy. A steady energy source will help ensure you are energized throughout the day. Fats prove to be a better fuel for the brain and the body.

5. It can help control hunger.

Fats do not only serve as a reliable energy source. It can also keep you feeling full for a much longer time than carbs can.

6. Keto can help in the treatment of epilepsy.

A ketogenic diet can help people suffering from epilepsy by lowering their medication needs. The diet provides an excellent way of controlling the condition. Otherwise, it won't be used for the treatment of epilepsy. In fact, it has been in use and has been producing great results for epilepsy sufferers since the 1900s. Until today, the ketogenic diet is widely used as a therapy for children, especially those with uncontrolled epilepsy.

7. It can help regulate cholesterol level and blood pressure.

The ketogenic diet promises weight loss results. Since blood pressure is associated with extra weight and keto can help manage weight, it can help with blood pressure problems as a result. Moreover, studies have shown that a low carb high fat diet can help in increasing HDL levels and decreasing LDL particle concentration. This is a positive note on account of managing your cholesterol level and also blood pressure.

8. It can help lower insulin resistance.

As you have learned in the previous chapters, high insulin resistance is bad. If insulin resistance is left unmanaged, it can easily lead to type II diabetes. A ketogenic diet however, can help lower insulin resistance and bring it down to a healthy range. This makes a keto diet excellent for pre-diabetics.

9. Keto can help control acne breakouts.

This low carb diet can not only help you get into shape. It can also improve your skin!

What to Avoid on a Ketogenic Diet

On this diet, you have to restrict your carb intake. Ideally, it should be limited to 15 grams a day. Carbs obtained from vegetables, dairy and nuts are alright.

However, it is best to avoid refined carbohydrates, starch and fruits with the exception of berries, star fruit and avocado. These fruits can be consumed but always in moderation. Here's a general list of what you should avoid on a low carb high fat diet.

- Sugar including maple syrup, agave, honey, etc.

- Fruits such as oranges, apple, banana, etc.

- Tubers including yams, potato, etc.

- Grains like cereal, rice, corn, wheat, etc.

What to EAT on a Keto Diet

A ketogenic diet is low in carbs, moderate in protein and high in fats. Your intake should follow this pie.

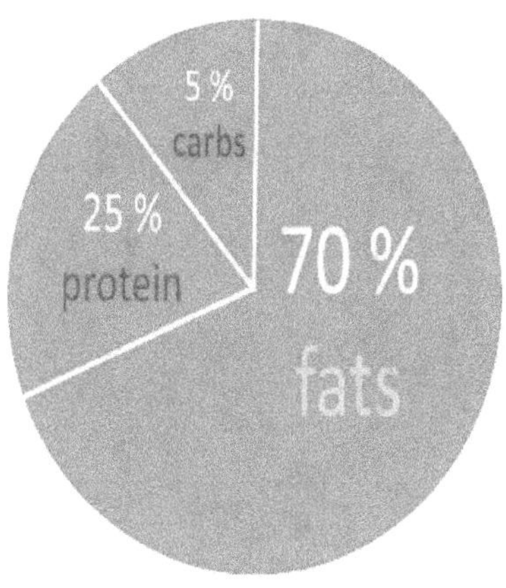

As an example, here is a list of what you should be chowing down on following a ketogenic diet.

- High Fat Dairy such as butter, high fat cream, hard cheeses, etc.

- Other fats including coconut oil, saturated fats, high-fat salad dressing, etc.

- Avocado and berries

- Nuts and seeds

- Protein meat sources like beef, lamb, fish, poultry, eggs, etc.

- Leafy green vegetables

- Above ground vegetables

Low carb sweeteners like monk fruit, stevia and erythritol are also allowed in moderation.

Why am I telling you all of this?

It is simply because it's good for you to know! Yes, you can proceed with intermittent fasting as it is and not think about what you eat. However, you will probably agree that making better food choices can do you more good than harm. So on your feasting periods, you may want to start thinking about what you eat. I promise, it doesn't take that much effort.

For instance, if you're used to having burgers or sandwich for lunch, you can simply take the bun or bread out of the equation. What's left is essentially keto!

If you're interested, you can check out my other book, "Keto for Beginners: Essentials to Get Started with the Ketogenic Diet and Reset Your Metabolism

in 14 Days."

Chapter 10
Ten-Day Meal Plan

Although intermittent fasting is a no-diet diet, this should not stop you from making healthier food choices. Ideally, your meal should have vegetables, protein and fats.

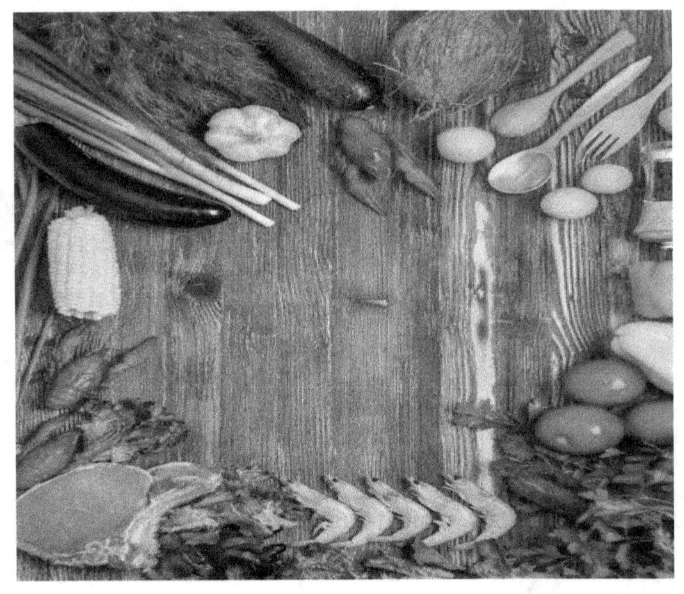

Make your meals more colorful!

URL Source:

https://www.pexels.com/photo/vegetables-and-tomatoes-on-cutting-board-255501/

How to serve your veggies!

Now, not everyone is a fan of vegetables. If your vocabulary on preparing veggies is a bit limited, here are a few ideas on how to make colorful vegetables much more interesting.

-Roast sweet potatoes, sprouts, cauliflower and broccoli. Don't forget to season them with salt and pepper.

-Wrap them in meat! For instance, asparagus wrapped in a half slice of prosciutto, spray with extra virgin olive oil and bake it. Another idea is wrapping two to three asparagus pieces in bacon and let it fry in bacon fat.

-Steam anything from peppers, cauliflower, asparagus, broccoli, onion, carrots and whatever you can find.

-You can also French fry thin slices of parsnips, carrots and sweet potatoes.

-Skewer and barbecue peppers, onion, zucchini and baby tomatoes. Marinade them in olive oil and season with salt and pepper.

-Turn them to rice or pasta! You can toss cauliflower in a blender and stir-fry to make cauliflower rice. You can also shred zucchini for a mock-up pasta.

-Make a smoothie out of your leafy greens. If you can't eat them, perhaps you can drink them. Smoothies are a great encouraging way to boost your leady green vegetables intake. Just do it gradually though.

Add variety to protein.

When you hear about protein, meat is probably the first thing that comes to your mind. You have beef, pork, chicken, ham, lamb, turkey, bison, etc. Don't be limited by the meats you are familiar with. You can go darker. Dark meats are usually packed with more flavor so it will be a good idea to try them out. Also, do not be afraid to explore ground meat options. When you're fasting, you have to make sure you enjoy your meals and are completely satisfied. Variety is great so keep exploring your options.

Don't forget your seafood. They're tasty and a lot of things can be done with them. Do not get stuck with tuna. Try salmon, mussels, shrimp, scallops, etc.

Another great protein source are dairy products. Eggs works not just for breakfast. If you're skipping the first meal of the day, you can always have your favorite egg breakfast meal for lunch. You can even have breakfast for dinner. Do whatever you like. Other dairy protein sources are Greek and goat yogurt, milk, ricotta and cottage cheese among others. Make sure you have a variety of these sources throughout the week.

More Fats!

Forget about what you were told about how fat can ruin your figure. Have butter! Think of cheese recipes. Use olive oil but not for frying. Get loads of nuts and seeds. Try out coconut and coconut oil. And please don't forget your avocado!

Assuming you're pulling a 16:8 protocol, here is a simple sample meal plan for you. Remember, you can have a glass of water or a cup of tea during your fasting period. A cup of coffee is also allowed as long as there is no cream or sugar in it.

Day One

Breakfast: A cup of coffee or tea

Lunch: Turkey sandwich

Dinner: Chili

Day Two

Breakfast: A cup of coffee or tea

Lunch: Chicken salad

Dinner: Grilled Salmon with side vegetables

Day Three

Breakfast: A cup of coffee or tea

Lunch: Mushroom bacon skillet

Dinner: Roasted chicken with side vegetables

Day Four

Breakfast: A cup of coffee or tea

Lunch: Asparagus wrapped in bacon with poached egg

Dinner: Creamy mushroom chicken

Day Five

Breakfast: A cup of coffee or tea

Lunch: Turkey Sausage Frittata

Dinner: Meatballs

Day Six

Breakfast: A cup of coffee or tea

Lunch: Stir-Fried shrimp with Cauliflower Rice

Dinner: White turkey chili

Day Seven

Breakfast: A cup of coffee or tea

Lunch: Tuna salad

Dinner: Pulled barbecue and roasted vegetables

Day Eight

Breakfast: A cup of coffee or tea

Lunch: Quinoa salad

Dinner: Chicken curry

Day Nine

Breakfast: A cup of coffee or tea

Lunch: Burrito bowl

Dinner: Roasted turkey with avocado tomato salad

Day Ten

Breakfast: A cup of coffee or tea

Lunch: Chickpea salad

Dinner: Buffalo chicken with Caesar salad

Just a tip! So you don't miss breakfast too much, you can have your favorite breakfast meals and recipes for lunch instead.

500-Calorie Meal Suggestions

If you're choosing the 5:2 protocol, here are a few ideas on 500-calorie meals.

-Baked cod in creamy tomato sauce

-Seared scallop in curry sauce with tart apples, dried cranberries and almonds

-Taco lettuce wraps

-Spinach salad with sliced beets, shredded carrots, hard-boiled eggs and blue cheese dressing

Conclusion

I'd like to thank you and congratulate you for transiting my lines from start to finish.

I hope this book was able to help you obtain a much deeper understanding about intermittent fasting and its incredible health benefits.

The next step is to create a new habit with IF in your routine! Remember to eat like an adult, eat slowly, drink plenty of water and keep an open mind. Be patient and monitor your progress.

I would like to remind you again that intermittent fasting is not a magic bullet. There is much to be expected from it but it requires your patience. Listen

to your body. Do not expect for miracles.

I wish you the best of luck!

www.ingramcontent.com/pod-product-compliance
Lightning Source LLC
Chambersburg PA
CBHW070122260726